INTRODUCTION

Anyone who believes that the appearance of a few strands of white hair indicates that it is time to stop is entirely mistaken.

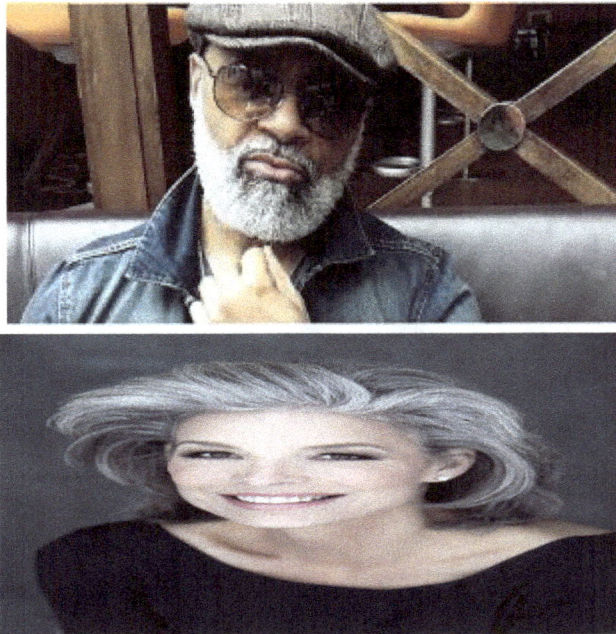

The assumption that you have made the most of your life by the age of 60 is far from true, and many people take advantage of the less hectic era of their lives to seek new experiences and pursue new dreams.

The golden years begin at the age of 65 and continue until the age of 80 or beyond, but finding methods to enjoy life as an elderly person is much easier than you might believe.

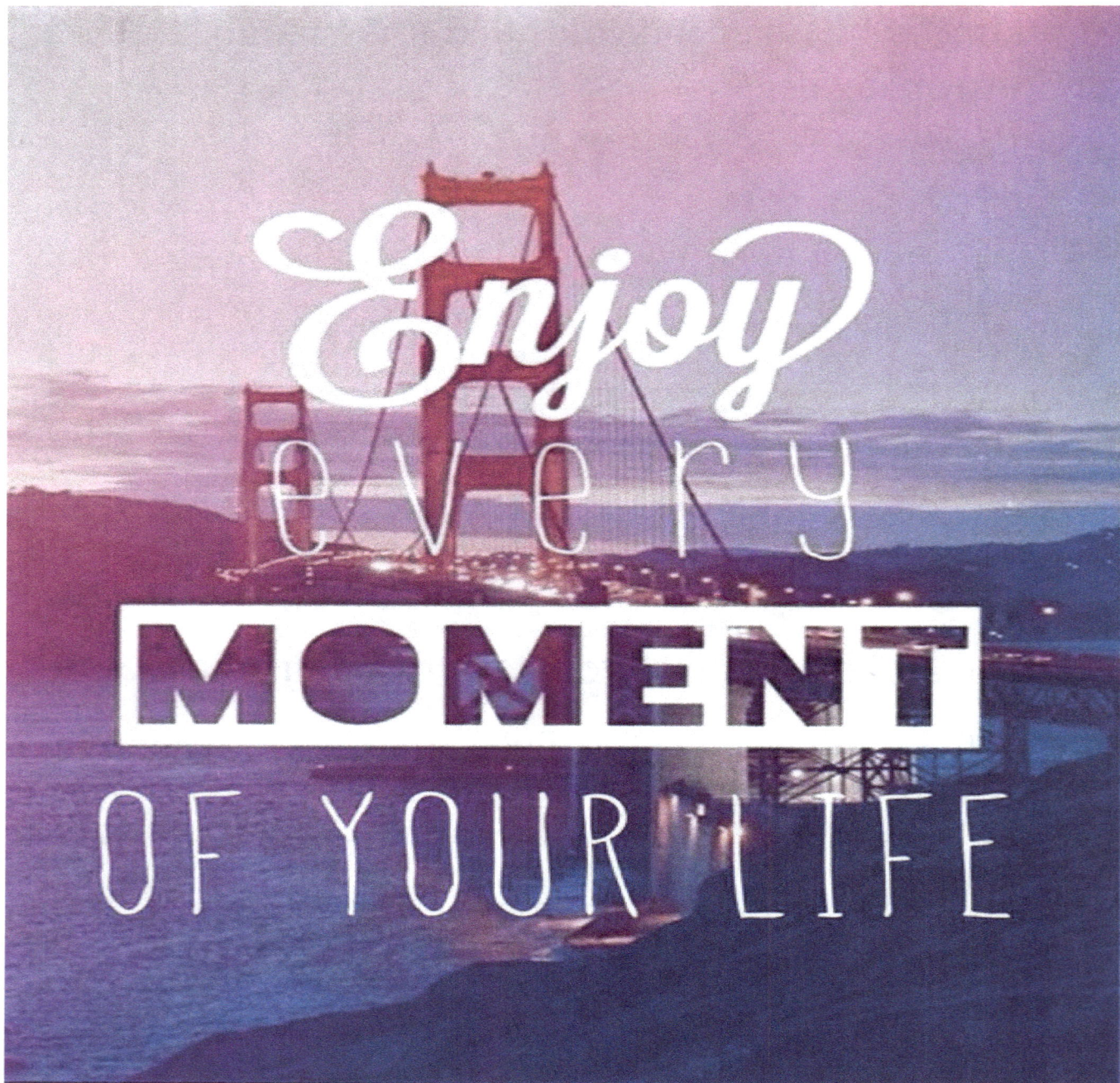

Of course, happiness varies greatly from person to person and at any age, but this stage of life can be really enjoyable! Time is no longer an issue; all you need to do is be willing and open to new learning and experiences.

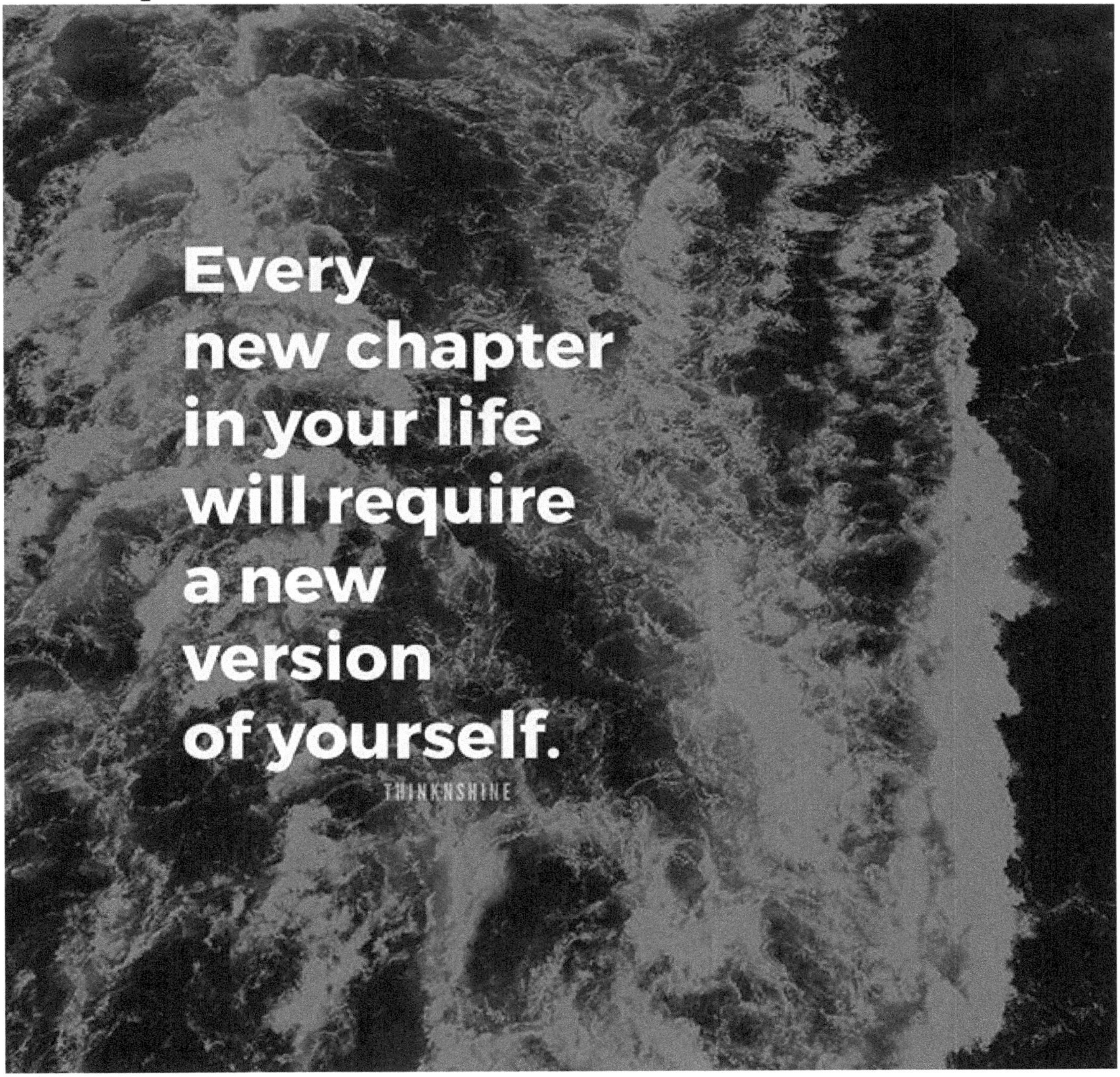

Every
new chapter
in your life
will require
a new
version
of yourself.

THINKNSHINE

Don't get me wrong: time does impose constraints on the body, but that doesn't mean you can't adjust to and welcome this new and exciting chapter of life.

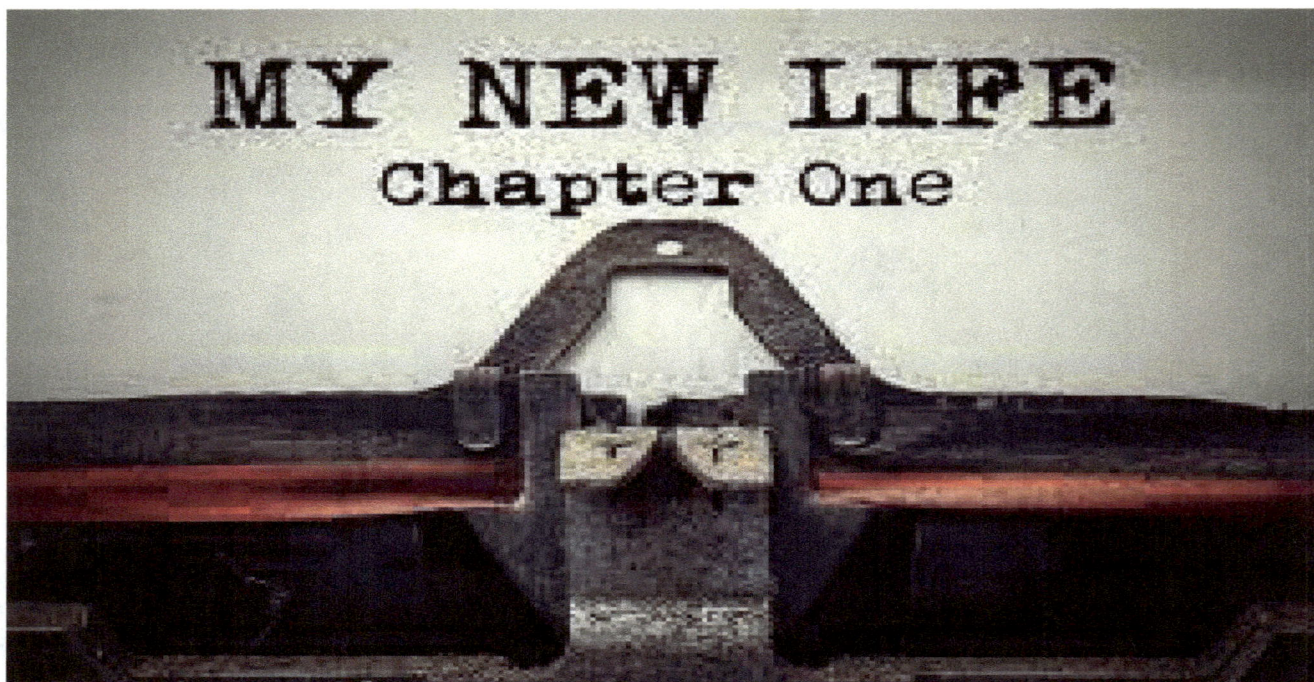

And how are you going to do it? A simple idea is to avoid becoming a victim of your age.

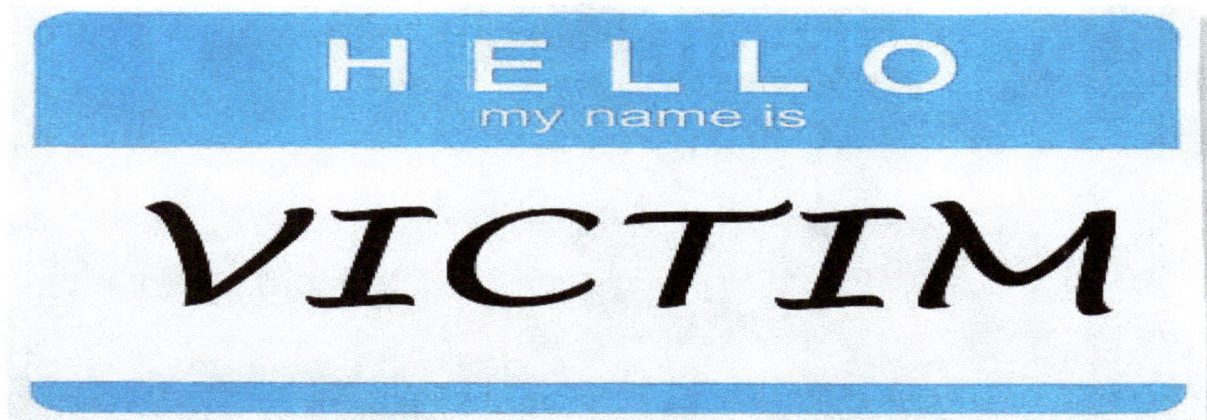

As a senior, you can do almost everything you did as a young adult, although with a little more prudence. Now that you have extra time, you can devote it to activities that bring you joy. Special moments with family, delicious food, leisure activities, physical activities, sports, learning, and (as bizarre as it may seem) immersion into the technological world are all interesting measures in your journey toward a happier life.

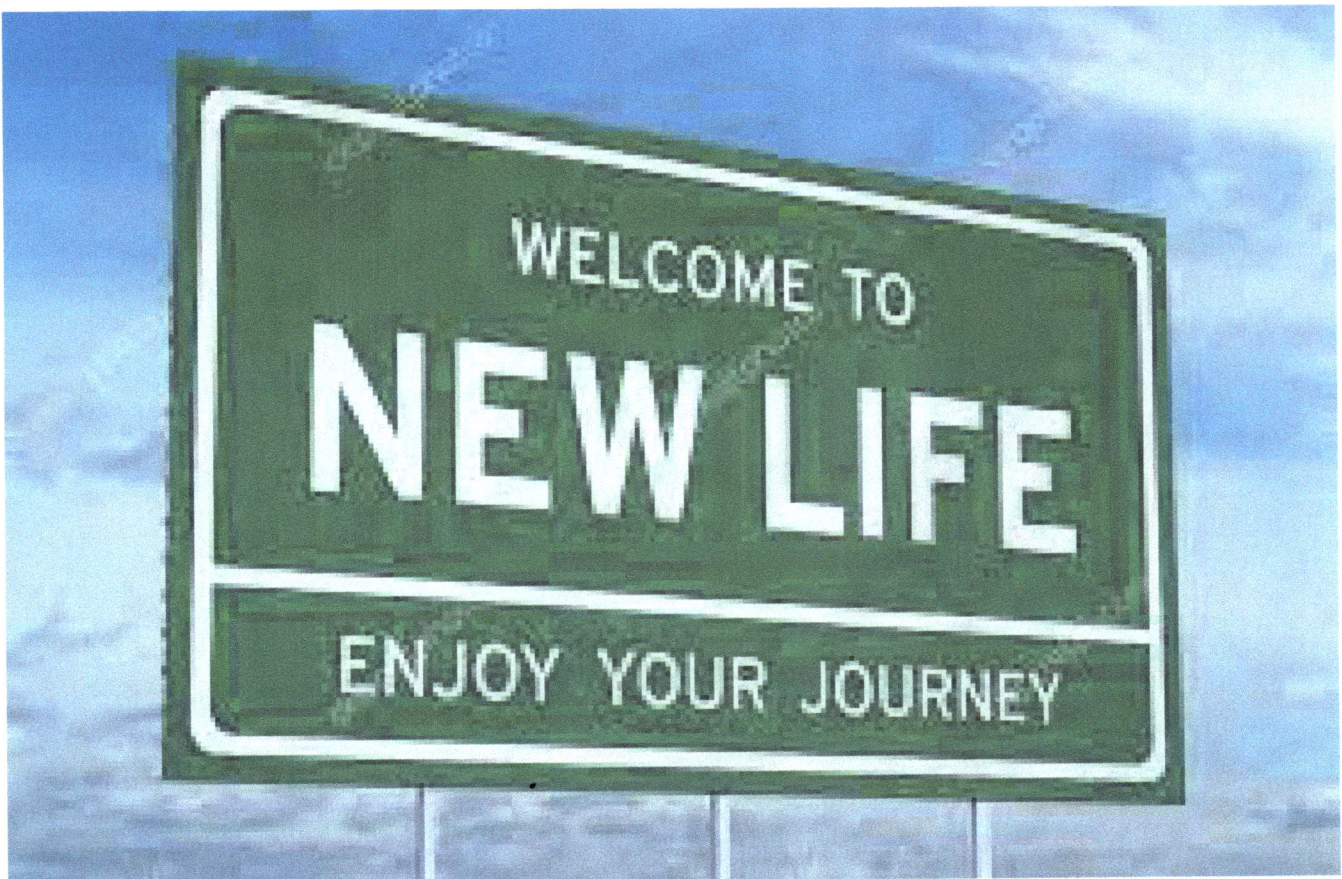

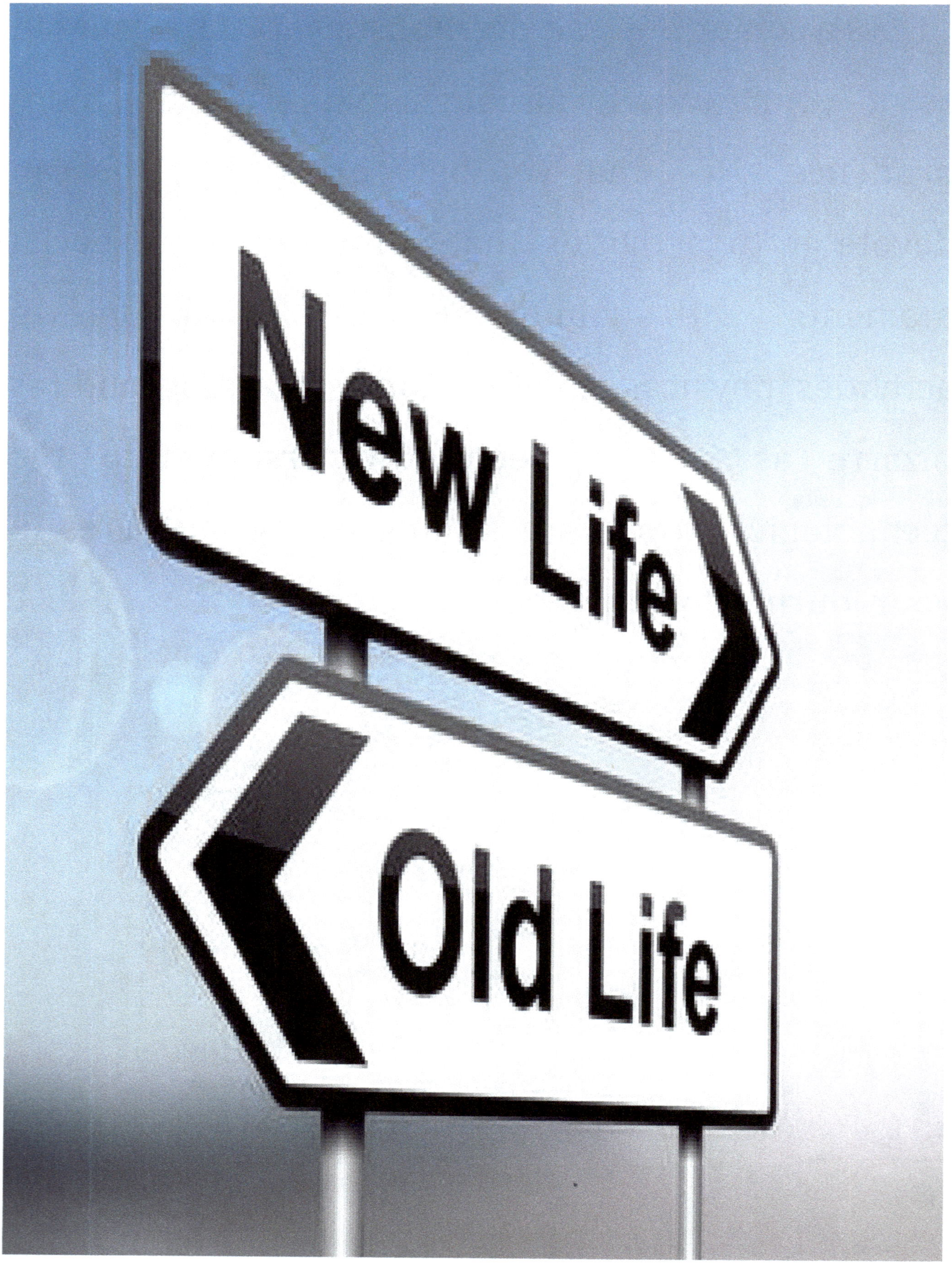

Finally, once you realize there are so many options, you'll be excited about what's to come. In this book, we'll go over some easy yet effective ways to make your golden years the finest of your life.

WELCOME TO YOUR BEST LIFE...

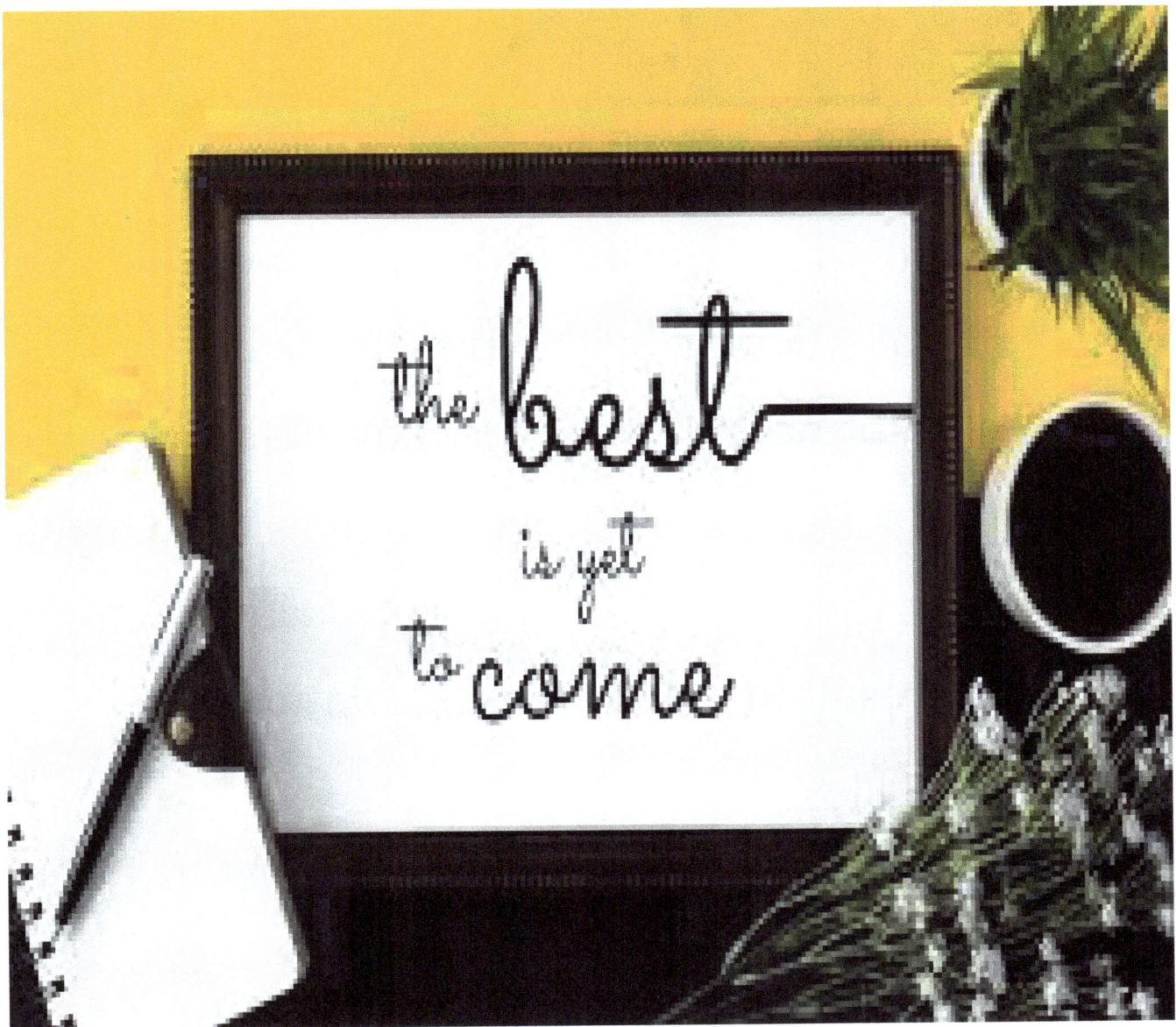

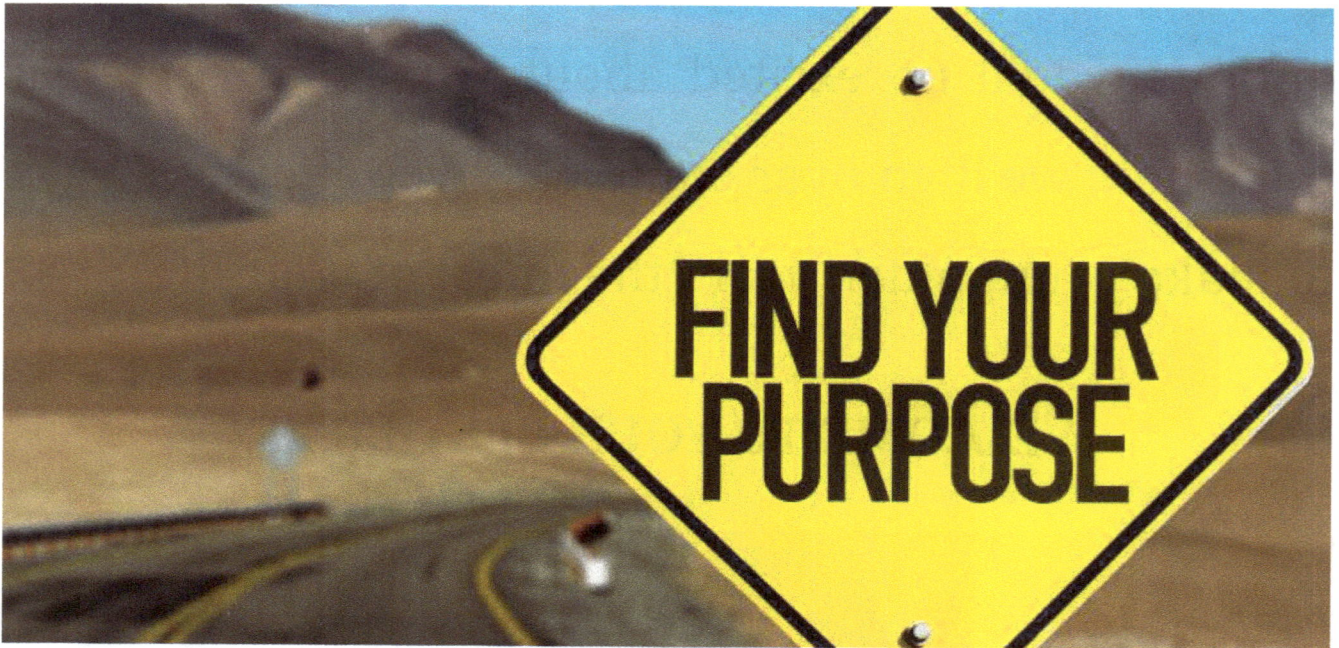

As you no longer deal with the day-to-day issues at work and the majority of people have finished most kinds of studying by this time in their lives, you run the risk of no longer having any objectives and purposes to follow or seek after retirement. Additionally, there is a decrease in social interaction, which may result in unintentional isolation.

In this context, setting some goals to pursue with the time available after retiring is a great way to have an active and social life and encourage socialization, as the tendency is to look for other people who have the same aspirations. Finding a purpose at this age can be the turning point for an improved quality of life, and it's never too late to find "the thing" that makes you excited to wake up in the morning.

Make a list of new places to visit or movies to watch; learn to dance or play some sport; participate in games like chess and checkers championships; start volunteering at your local shelter or retirement home; you can even open a new business! Although these are just a few examples of how to find purposeful and more pleasant activities to do, they are great options to incorporate small and attainable foals into your routine. Focus on things that are a bit challenging but also doable.

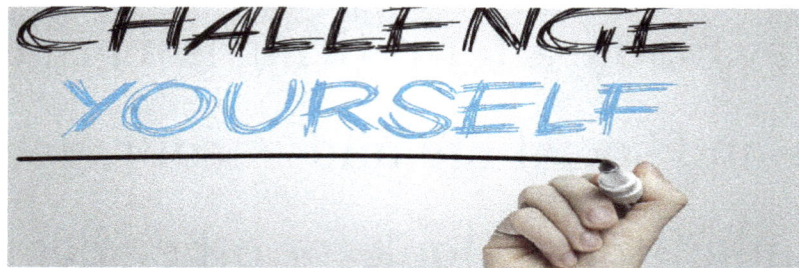

Make sure to always have many options listed as well. The lack of goals or even the achievement of them without the existence of a new one can cause a feeling of emptiness capable of leading to a lack of emotional balance. So, keep your hands full! It is never too late to have a purposeful and fulfilling life.

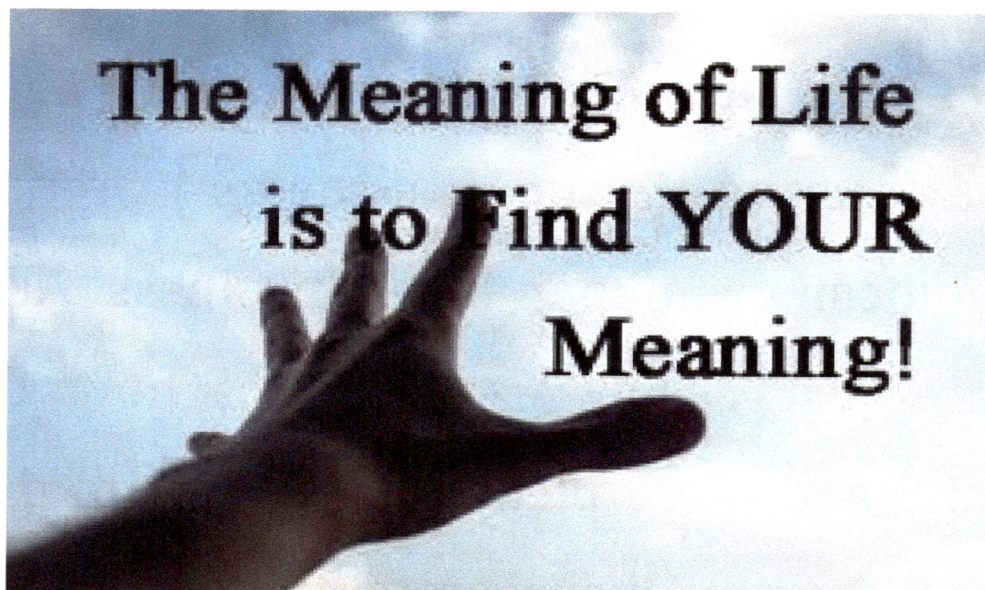

PART 02. HEALTH IN THE GOLDEN AGE.

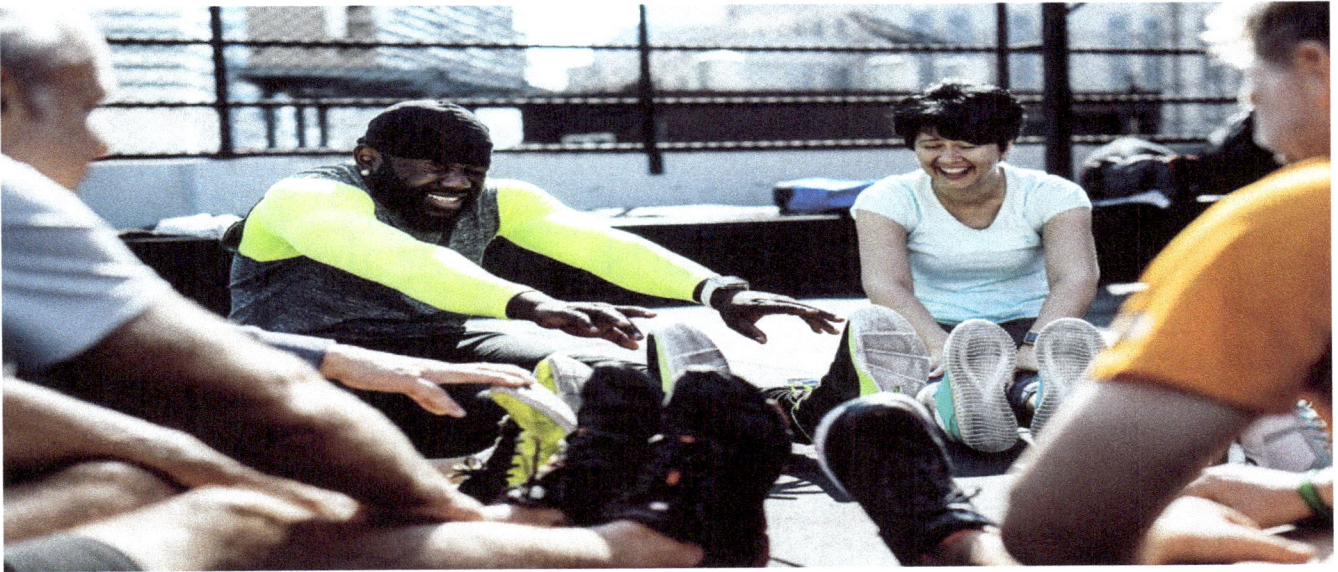

We are all aware of the necessity of maintaining our health at any age, but it is evident that advanced age demands a bit more of our attention. Physical exercise is not just a technique to avoid obesity and lower the risk of developing diseases such as hypertension and diabetes; it is also how our bodies release endorphins, one of the hormones responsible for feelings of joy and well-being. Thus, helping to avoid depression and anxiety.

In addition, muscle strengthening is essential at this stage of life to ensure an active and independent life. Thus, preserving the ability to perform everyday actions, such as bathing and dressing alone. The idea is to exercise at least 3 times a week. Also, activities such as swimming, walking, and even weight training - if there is no medical contraindication - help to maintain body mass and, when well oriented, do not harm bones and joints.

Another important measure to make the most of the golden age and ensure that this is a phase of great vitality is to create the habit of doing simple activities daily that exercise the brain, stimulating short and long-term memory and increasing focus and concentration.

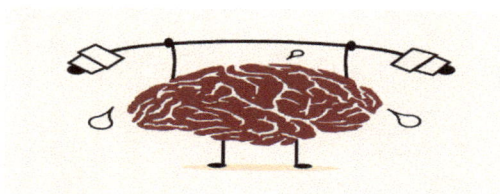

You can, for example, dedicate your time to solving a crossword puzzle, which helps to improve cognitive functions, or stimulate the senses with different activities, such as discovering a new musical style or trying a dish from an unknown cuisine. The practice of such games that require the solving of a problem, such as word searches, and sudoku, among others, is also a very pleasant way to keep the mind active while also having a lot of fun.

Another interesting possibility in this context is to dedicate some time to games that require concentration instead, such as cards and chess, or to reading, which, in addition to exercising the brain, also helps to keep vocabulary memory intact.

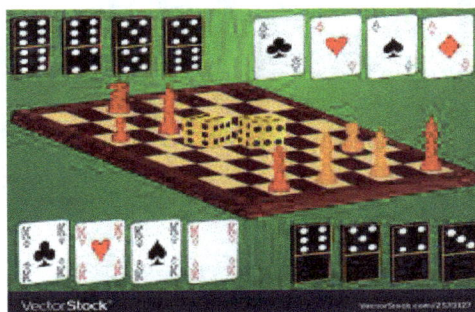

Also, try to help others with their problems and give advice!

A brain used to solve problems is much more likely to stay healthy. Therefore, solving day-to-day issues will keep your mind active and give you a sense of belonging, which is so important at any stage of life.

PART 03. REMAINING SOCIAL

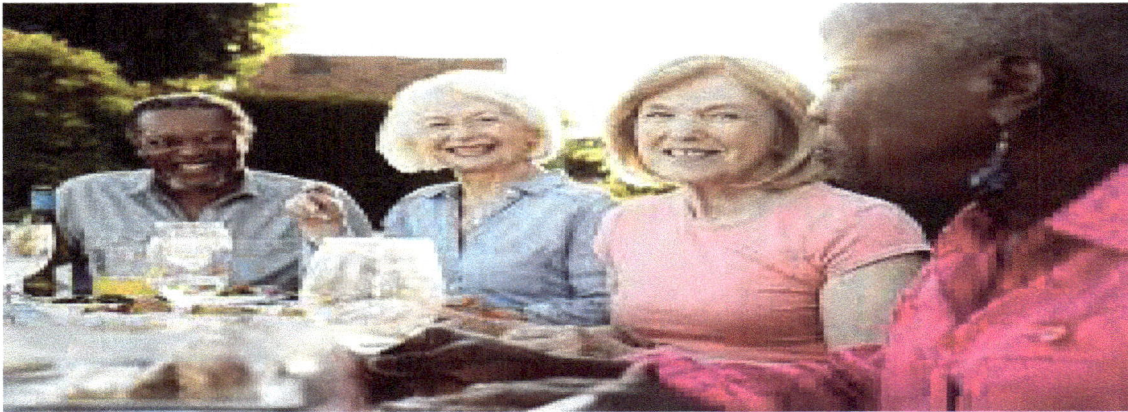

We've seen how to keep your body and mind active with games and workouts in the previous section, but just as essential as taking care of our physical and mental health by doing things alone is making sure we're also surrounded by people we love.

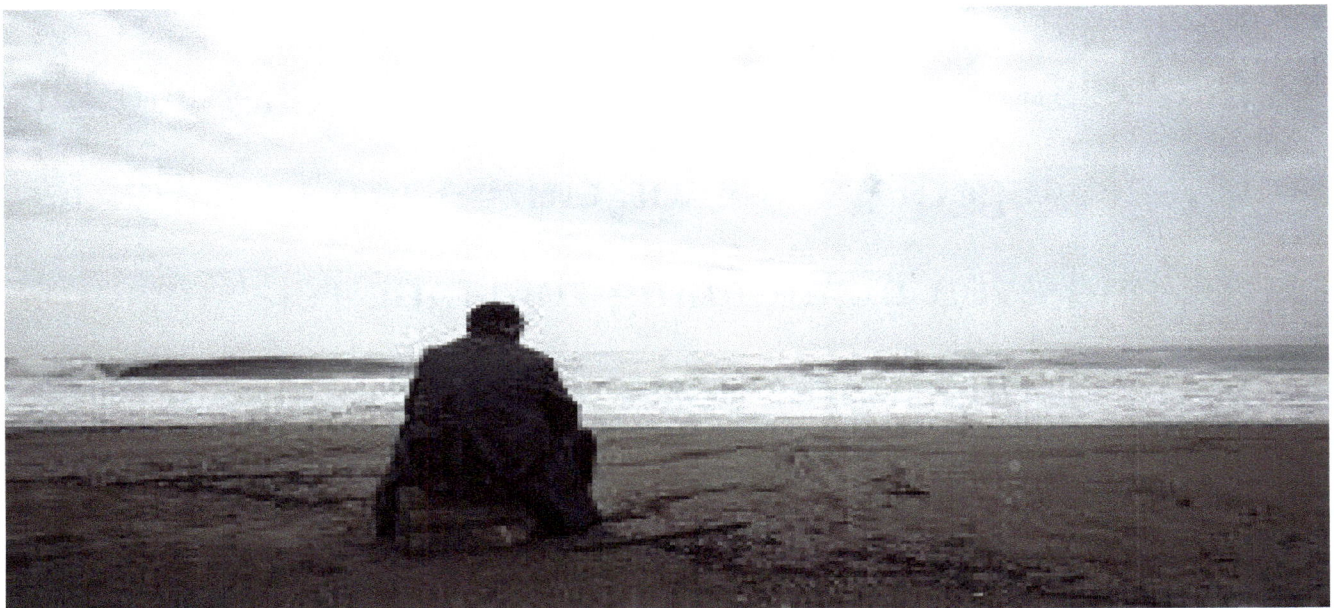

Feeling alone and disconnected from others, especially family and friends, is one of the worst things that may happen at this age. And it is common for people with mobility disabilities to end up depending primarily on visitation.

This means that social interaction is necessary to avoid feeling lonely and developing depressive symptoms.

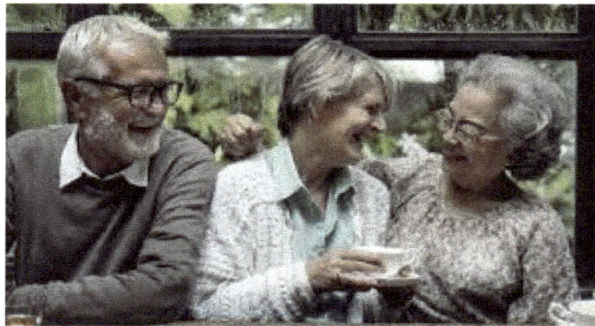

Make sure to have a busy social life, including family get-togethers, senior citizen group activities, travel, and even maintaining romantic relationships. These activities support greater enjoyment and well-being while reducing stress, relieving pain, and boosting the immune system.

Additionally, maintaining social connections lowers the chance of cardiovascular disease development and aids in maintaining cognitive abilities, particularly memory.

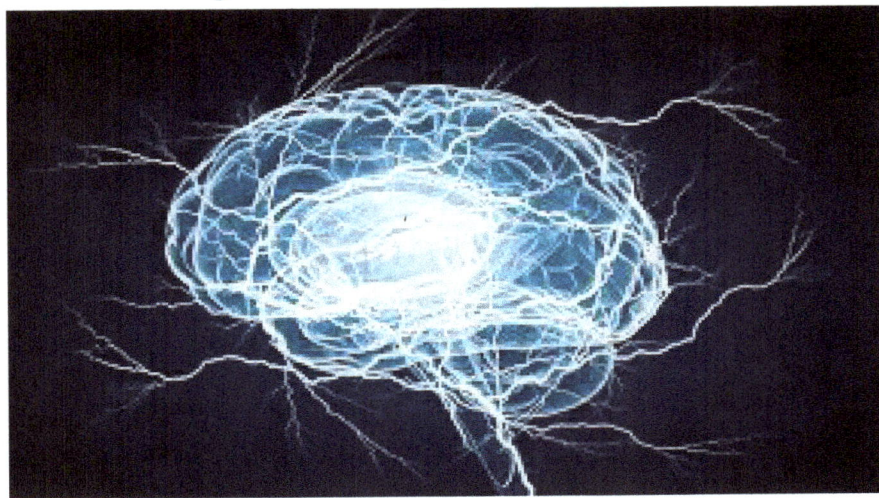

If you have limited mobility, such as being bedridden or hospitalized, it is important for your family to organize a routine of constant visits and for you to always have a trusted person nearby, such as a caregiver or family member living in the same neighborhood.

This aspect ensures that you'll not feel alone and that you'll receive the necessary help in unexpected day-to-day situations that you're unable to deal with.

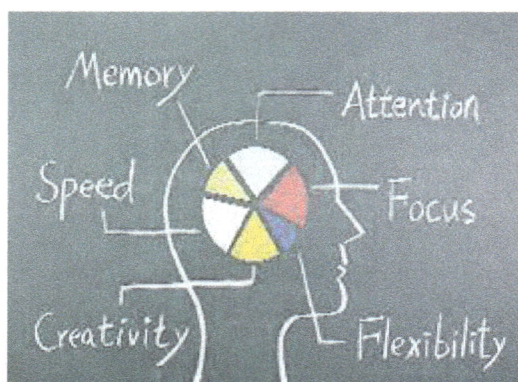

And if you still don't have any mobility limitations, it is important to encourage yourself to socialize with other people who have common interests. Go out there and try to be part of a group of some sort.

It can be a book club, a traveling team, etc. This will not only improve your sense of belonging and keep your mind and body healthier and active but will also drastically improve your quality of life.

PART 04. FINDING JOY IN THE SMALLEST THINGS.

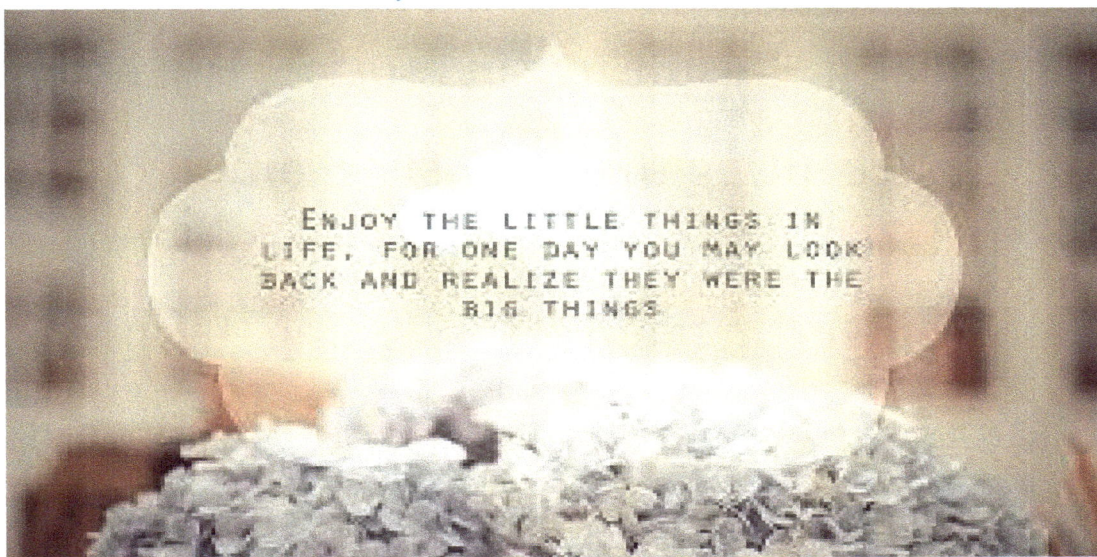

ENJOY THE LITTLE THINGS IN LIFE, FOR ONE DAY YOU MAY LOOK BACK AND REALIZE THEY WERE THE BIG THINGS.

Many seniors suffer from low self-esteem issues, and most of the time, it is about more than simply appearance; it is also about a person's lifestyle. It is normal for older people, for example, to feel like a burden or worthless.

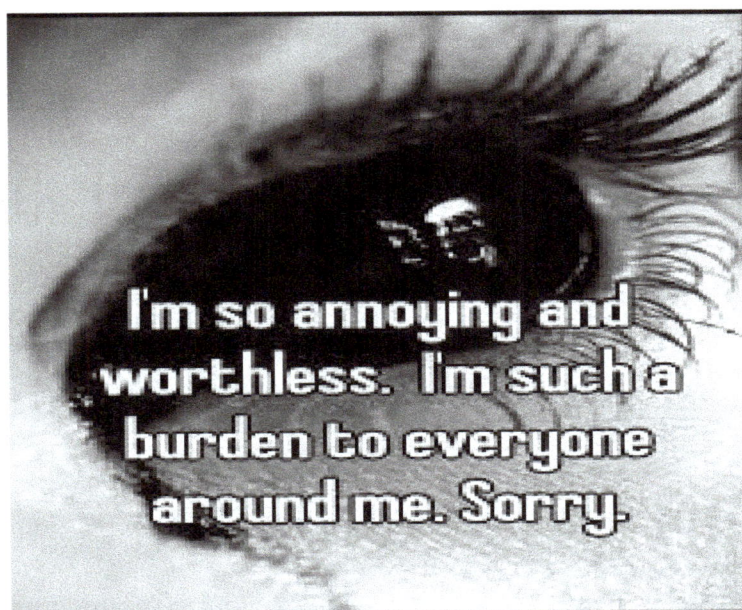

I'm so annoying and worthless. I'm such a burden to everyone around me. Sorry.

This has an impact on both psychological and physical health, resulting in social isolation and difficulty in accepting this new chapter.

Afraid of getting old or wanting to prevent it from happening, you can end up failing to enjoy the small moments of this phase or even prepare for it financially.

In the end, struggling to accept the moment for what it is will prevent you from fully enjoying what the golden age has to offer. And the result could not be other than a lack of quality of life.

Even though aging is totally natural, western society nevertheless views it in a distorted light, as if it must be avoided. This is what causes people to want to look young all the time or to be unwilling to deal with this phase of life. However, in order to make your golden years the greatest of your life, you must approach aging in the best way possible, viewing it as a period in which new discoveries and experiences can still happen.

It's true that seniors require specific attention in many ways, but many people get carried away, lacking any motivation to experience something new or take care of their own health. However, this phase in our lives is all about small pleasures, and seniors should celebrate their own accomplishments! By noticing, for example, that the years lived provided you with a very valuable perspective, you might begin to appreciate what you have lived thus far and what the coming years may bring.

Recognize that growing older does not imply the end of your life. Things change, but there is still a way to appreciate new experiences, discover new goals, and even fulfill ambitions. That is why it is critical to seek out new ways to enjoy your days, whether through new hobbies or through simply doing what you enjoy. The goal is to uncover new ways to learn that this stage can be quite meaningful.

Look for new habits that will keep your daily life interesting and meaningful. Plant and care for a garden in your backyard on a daily basis, do DIY projects to decorate and personalize your space, play games, read, talk, and laugh a lot, and focus on living life to the fullest rather than worrying about making or spending more money! Most importantly, spend quality time with those you care about and fill your days with activities that make you happy.

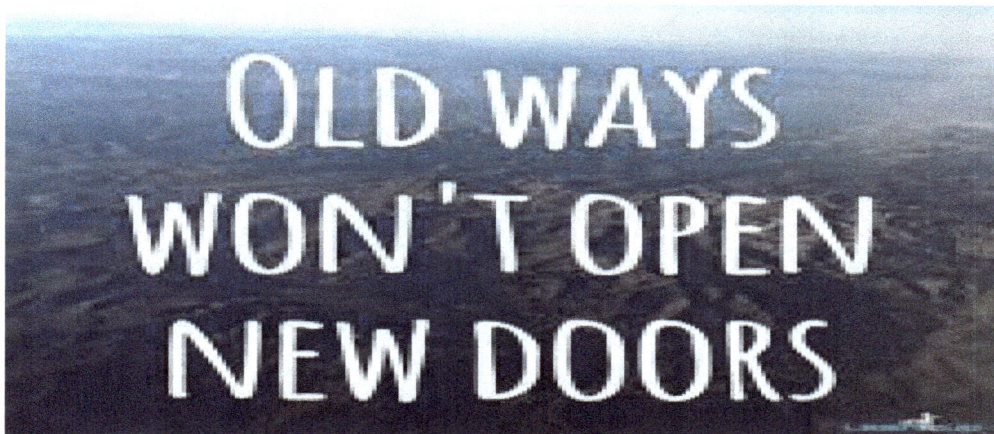

OLD WAYS WON'T OPEN NEW DOORS

We've all heard great stories about people who achieved early success in business and in life. At the age of 19, Mark Zuckerberg founded Facebook. At the age of 21, Steve Jobs established Apple. Warren Buffett is even more astounding... he started investing at the age of seven when he asked his father for a book on government bonds as a Christmas present.

Then you hear these stories about young geniuses and decide that at 25, you're too old to turn your life around and start chasing your dreams. You believe that changing your life at 30 is impossible, that starting a new career at 40 is unattainable, and that after you reach your 50s, 60s, 70s, and even 80s, you're essentially done with life and must live it at home watching Animal Planet.

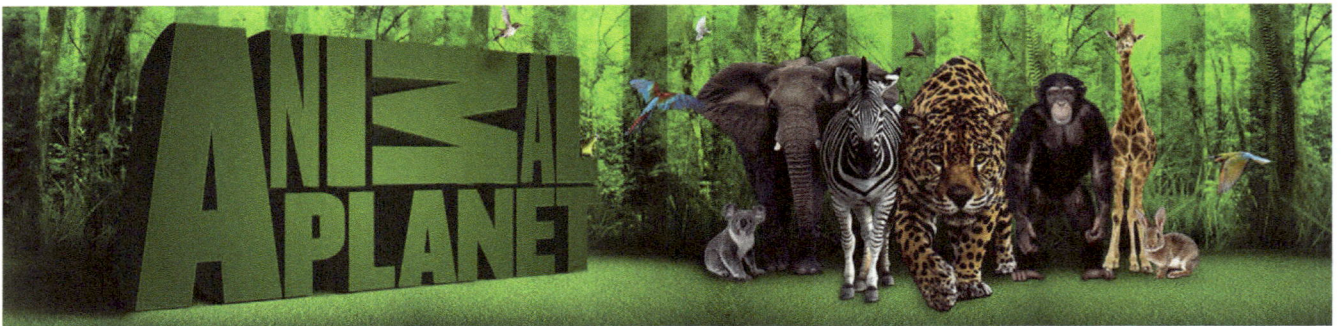

You're wrong! Any obstacle you imagine you have is, in fact, just and entirely in your mind, and it is easily eliminated with the right attitudes and beliefs. Stop thinking you're "past your prime."

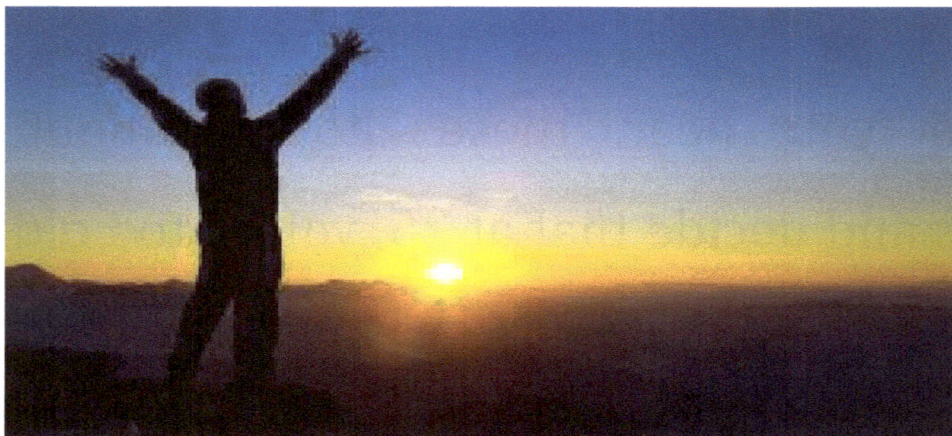

Believe it or not, just as there are stories of people who "made it" when they were still kids, there are equally as many stories of people who achieved success close to their golden age. Let me give you a few examples:

John Pemberton developed the most recognizable brand in the world and possibly of all time. Yes, I'm talking about Coca-Cola. And anyone who believes the concept has been developed since his youth is mistaken. Actually, his invention was the result of his ideas upon his return from the American Civil War in 1886, when he was 55 years old.

Because Facebook, Instagram, and Apple were founded by extremely young individuals, many people believe that the greatest digital ideas come from very young people, practically teens. But they're also wrong! As an example, Jan Koum and Brian Acton, 35 and 37 years old, invented WhatsApp, which was recently purchased by Facebook for an astounding sum of $16 billion.

In short, you don't have to be better or younger than anyone else to be successful in your life. Get the idea of comparing yourself to others out of your head.

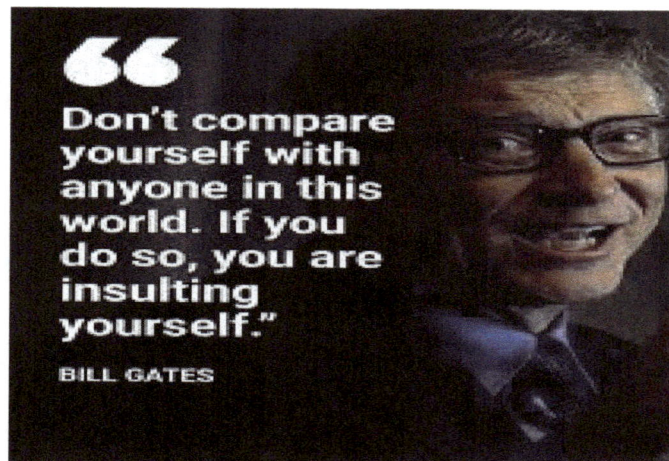

Don't compare yourself with anyone in this world. If you do so, you are insulting yourself."

BILL GATES

Each person has a different story and, therefore, different goals to achieve in life. And to achieve your goals, whatever they are, you don't have to look at others and regret not having started sooner or try to be better than others.

If you haven't found anything that satisfies you until you're 30, 40, 50, 60, 70, 80, 90, or even 100, no problem! Keep looking. One day you will find it, and the moment you find it, don't be ashamed to go after what you want. As Steve Jobs said:

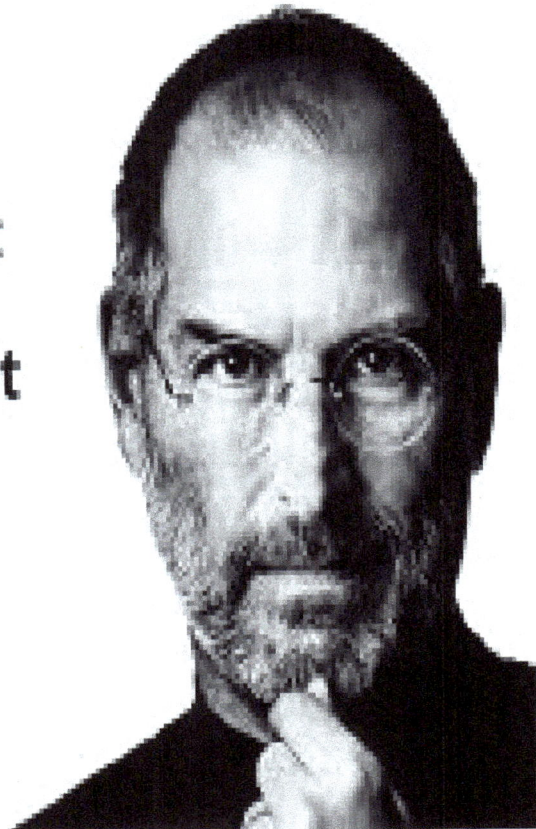

"Have the courage to follow your heart and intuition. They somehow know what you truly want to become."

- Steve Jobs

PART 06. BEING THANKFUL

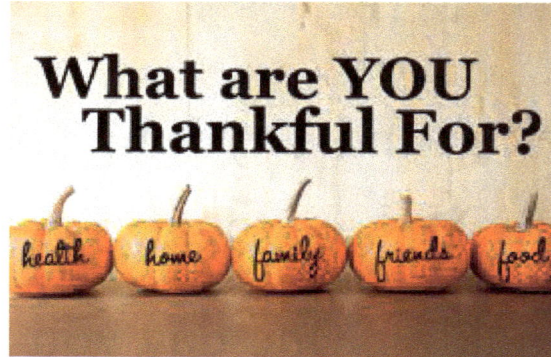

It's common to give thanks for everyday gestures, like when someone holds the elevator door, waiting for you to get in. But are we grateful for the prime of our lives and the years we've lived? How important is our gratitude? After all, getting older seems like a great idea when we consider the alternatives. In this sense, we need to realize that gratitude is what can make us feel lighter and at peace with ourselves.

Gratitude is something innate in human beings and even interferes with our brains. Every time we give thanks and feel grateful for something or someone, levels of dopamine, which, as we know, is a neurotransmitter responsible for well-being, mood, and pleasure, increase. Consequently, we feel happier, lighter, and more satisfied because we activate the brain's reward system.

The feeling of gratitude goes far beyond what we think is positive as well. It is more associated with a state of mind, as we can practice gratitude in relation to many different events. This means that we can also feel grateful in the face of experiences that we judge as negative, for example. We may have learned several lessons or, at the very least, found an opportunity for a fresh start. In the end, simply being alive and reaching the golden age in itself is a compelling reason to be thankful.

But how can we be more grateful? One of my favorite activities is the **Gratitude Notebook.**

Start with gratitude

Five-minute daily gratitude journal

This is already a well-known practice, and it is a notebook that should be kept by your bed, always accompanied by a pen or pencil. The intention is that, when you wake up or before you go to sleep, you write down 3-4 **things you are grateful for that day.**

It may be that, at first, there is some difficulty in listing all these reasons, but it's all about how you perceive things and situations. It's not about looking for stratospheric things. There are people who believe that they will only have real reasons to practice gratitude when they win the lottery, get promoted to the position of dreams, or find a prince charming. Instead, focus on the little things. Give thanks for your bed, for the comfortable pillow, for the clothes you are wearing, for your eyes, which allow you to see, for your mouth, which gives you the possibility to speak, for the food, for the hot bath...

In the end, the power of gratitude is real and can be applied by anyone, and it's also a way of appreciating all the people who still are or have passed through our lives – each one, in fact, matters! The more we put effort into understanding how to practice gratitude, the more our minds become attuned to its foundation as well. That is, we will be able to enjoy all the benefits it can provide. So, exercise the power of gratitude whenever you have the opportunity. Considering this an exercise as important as any other physical or mental activity!

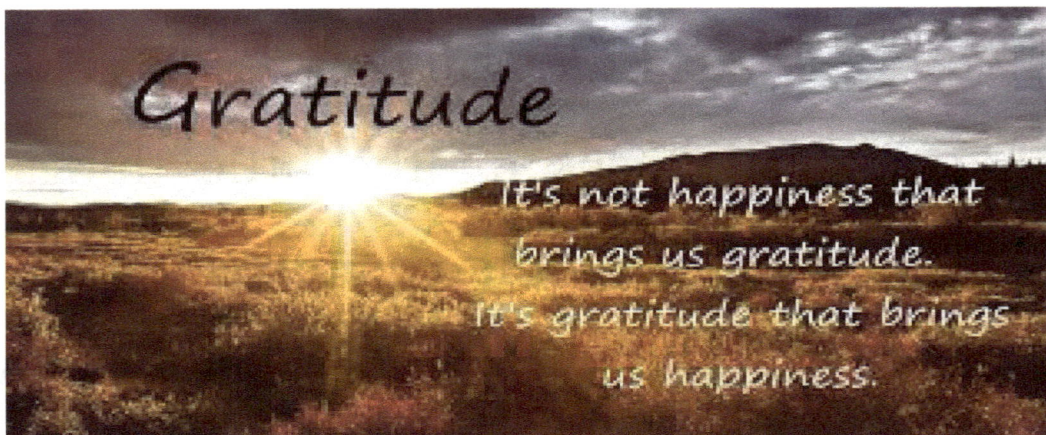

Gratitude

It's not happiness that brings us gratitude. It's gratitude that brings us happiness.

Despite being part of the natural cycle of life, many people are afraid of getting old, seeing it, in most cases, as a phase to be avoided or hidden. However, aging is natural and, despite the myths and stereotypes, there are several benefits that await us at this stage of life.

Achieving the golden age is an important milestone in our existence. It is a reflection of everything that we have lived and conquered in the previous age groups, and it should not, in any way, be seen as something negative. Taking into account the experience gained and the more relaxed lifestyle, it can even be considered one of the **best phases of our lives.**

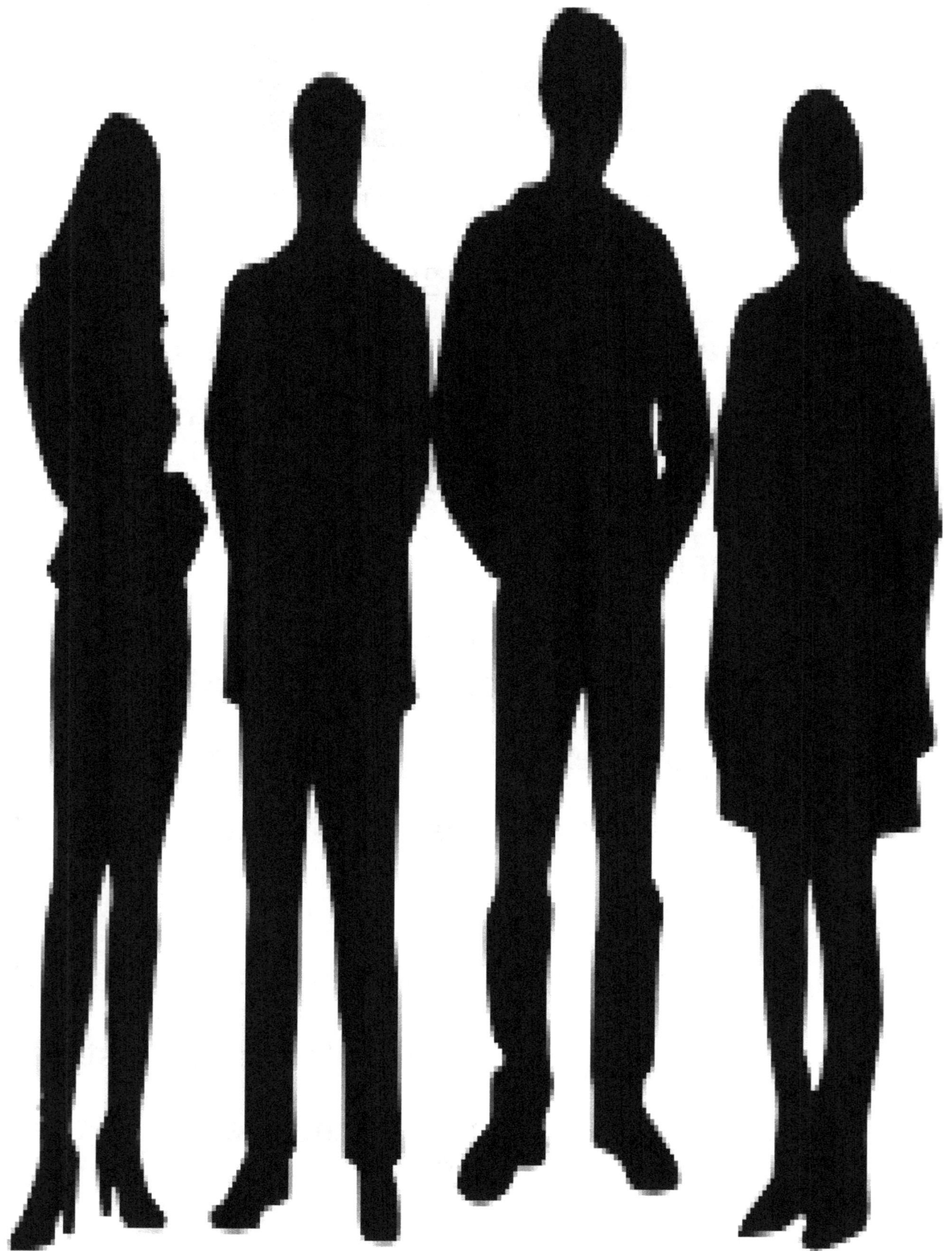

I hope the tips in this book help you improve your quality of life and ensure that your golden age is nothing but a fantastic and fulfilling new chapter of life.

Go Live Your Best Life...

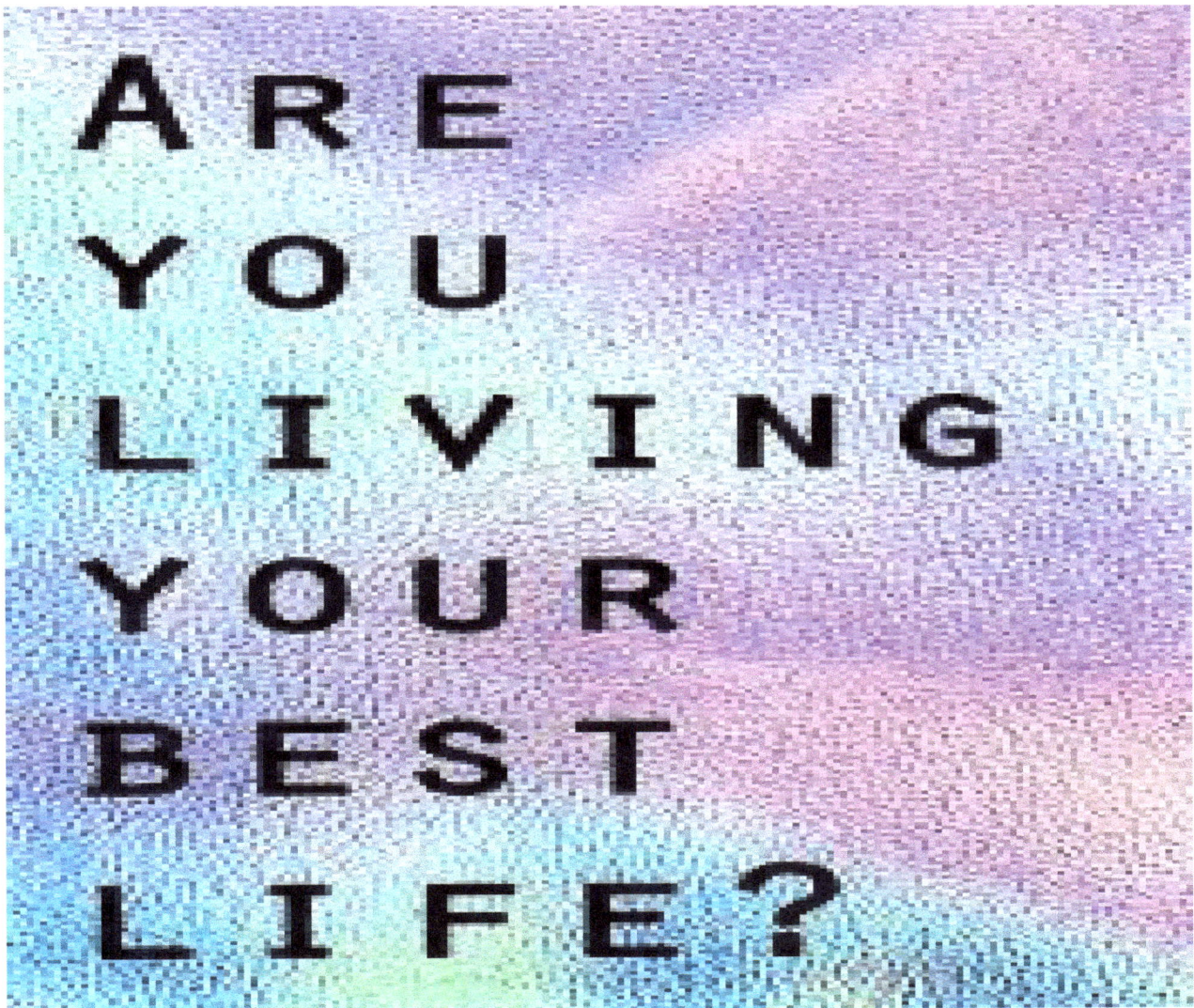
ARE YOU LIVING YOUR BEST LIFE?

Write your new goals.

www.ingramcontent.com/pod-product-compliance
Lightning Source LLC
Chambersburg PA
CBHW061959090426
42811CB00006B/992